CW00820114

Disclaimer

This book is intended to help people become bet
consumers. The information in this book is intended to supplement,
not replace, the medical advice of a trained health care professional.
No mention or description of uses of drugs listed herein should be
construed as an endorsement of those uses or drugs. Only a physician
can prescribe drugs and their precise dosages. All matters regarding your
health require medical supervision. The authors and publisher disclaim
any liability arising directly or indirectly from use of this book.

Notice of rights

Trademarks

Many of the designations used by manufacturers and sellers to
distinguish their products are claimed as trademarks. Where those
designations appear in this book, and the publisher was aware of a
trademark claim, the designations appear as requested by the owner
of the trademark. All other product names and services identified
throughout this book are used in editorial fashion only and for the
benefit of such companies with no intention of infringement of the
trademark. No such use, or the use of any trade name, is intended to
convey endorsement or other affiliation with this book.

Table of Contents

Your feedback is invaluable to us

If you recently bought this book, we would love to hear from you! You can do this by writing a review on amazon (or the online store where you purchased this book) about your last purchase! As part of our continual service improvement process, we love to hear real client experiences and feedback.

How does it work?
To post a review on Amazon, just log in to your account and click on the Create Your Own Review button (under Customer Reviews) of the relevant product page. You can find examples of product reviews in Amazon. If you purchased from another online store, simply follow their procedures.

Why use this book?

Everyone should ask questions when getting a prescription. This is especially important when your doctor or other health care professional prescribes you Chlorpromazine Hydrochloride.

What should you ask?

Your health depends on good communication, but which questions to ask your doctor? Having the right questions is the answer.

Asking questions and providing information to your doctor and other care providers can improve your care. Talking with your doctor builds trust and leads to better satisfaction, quality, safety and results.

Asking questions is key to good communication with your doctor. If you do not ask questions, he or she may assume you already know the answer or that you do not want more information. Do not wait for the doctor to raise a specific question or subject; he or she may not know it is important to you. Be proactive. Ask questions.

Effective health care is a team effort. You are part of this team and play an important role. One of the best ways to communicate with your doctor and health care team is by asking questions. Since time is limited when you have your medical appointments, you will feel less rushed when you prepare your questions before your appointment.

Your doctor wants your questions. Doctors know a lot about a lot of things, but they do not always know everything about you, what you want to know or what is best for you.

Your questions give your doctor and health care professionals important information about you, like your most important health care concerns.

That is why they need you to speak up.

How to use this book?

When you meet with your doctor or other members of your health care team, you will hear a lot of information. It helps to think ahead of time of the things you want to know and to highlight the questions in this book you want to ask and take this book with you to your appointments.

This book contains questions you may want to ask your doctor. You should use the questions that fit your situation, and skip those that do not apply.

This book offers many ways that you can ask questions and get your health care needs met. With this book you will have numerous simple questions that can help you take better care of yourself, feel better, and get the right care at the right time.

Doctors and medical professionals want to know your questions to help them take better care of you and offer advice to get your most pressing questions answered.

Be prepared for your next medical appointment. Take this book with you if you are getting a checkup, want to discuss a problem or health condition, are getting a prescription, or talk about a medical test or surgery and be sure to write down the answers your health care professional provides for you in this book.

Whatever the reason for your appointment, it is important to be prepared.

Take charge of your health. Ask your health care providers questions and learn about the Chlorpromazine Hydrochloride medicine you take.

BEGINNING OF THE QUESTION CHAPTERS:

CHAPTER #1: WHO:

INTENT: Who benefits from
Chlorpromazine Hydrochloride (Is this
right for me.)

1. Are side effects from Chlorpromazine Hydrochloride medications the same in males and females?

Notes:

2. Is there a possibility of reaction to Chlorpromazine Hydrochloride medications?

Notes:

3. Do you know all of the risks Chlorpromazine Hydrochloride prescription drugs might pose?

Notes:

4. What is the Prescription Drug Monitoring Database and who is using it?

Notes:

5. Who should NOT take Chlorpromazine Hydrochloride medication?

Notes:

6. How will I know when my Chlorpromazine Hydrochloride medications are working?

Notes:

7. How do you help someone who has a Chlorpromazine Hydrochloride prescription drugs addiction?

Notes:

8. Who can assist with Chlorpromazine Hydrochloride medication reminders?

Notes:

9. Should I be on Chlorpromazine Hydrochloride medication?

Notes:

10. Can my baby get harmed by my Chlorpromazine Hydrochloride prescription drug use?

Notes:

11. Are there other ways to treat my condition?

Notes:

12. How do you prevent re-admission in case I forget to take my Chlorpromazine Hydrochloride prescription medications. How do you help those who have problems following suggestions regarding eating habits, smoking, drinking, and taking drugs..?

Notes:

13. Are you considering a trial of Chlorpromazine Hydrochloride medications and/or anything else?

Notes:

14. So who approves these Chlorpromazine Hydrochloride medications?

Notes:

15. What kinds of medications will I need to take and what if they don't work?

Notes:

16. Who can join a Medicare Chlorpromazine Hydrochloride prescription drug plan?

Notes:

17. Is there an Over-The-Counter Medication that helps or maybe even can replace my Chlorpromazine Hydrochloride Prescription Medication?

Notes:

18. How can a wholesome mud-bath help my condition, and what is the effect on my Chlorpromazine Hydrochloride prescription drugs?

Notes:

19. How does a Chlorpromazine Hydrochloride medication reminder service work?

Notes:

20. Who gets Chlorpromazine Hydrochloride, and when?

Notes:

21. Could natural products be just as effective as Chlorpromazine Hydrochloride prescription medications?

Notes:

22. Should I review my Medicare prescription drug plan choice every year?

Notes:

23. Will I be on Chlorpromazine Hydrochloride medication forever?

Notes:

24. What if I am affected by anxiety and don't like the thought of taking prescription medications?

Notes:

25. Who is most susceptible to Chlorpromazine Hydrochloride prescription drug abuse?

Notes:

26. Who is qualified to receive Chlorpromazine Hydrochloride prescription drug help?

Notes:

27. Has there been any follow up of those who have stopped taking Chlorpromazine Hydrochloride medication?

Notes:

28. Is there any form of exercise or medication you can recommend to enhance the effects of Chlorpromazine Hydrochloride?

Notes:

29. What are the active ingredients in Chlorpromazine Hydrochloride prescription medication?

Notes:

30. Um - can you explain that again?

Notes:

31. Does my plan cover the Chlorpromazine Hydrochloride prescription drugs I need?

Notes:

32. Can my Chlorpromazine Hydrochloride medication be delivered if I don't attend appointments?

Notes:

33. Who is accountable for my Chlorpromazine Hydrochloride prescription drug use?

Notes:

34. Do younger people need less of the Chlorpromazine Hydrochloride medication than older people?

Notes:

35. Who can I contact if I want to meet with a specialist for long-term Chlorpromazine Hydrochloride medication management on an ongoing basis?

Notes:

36. Are all drug-drug interactions limited to Chlorpromazine Hydrochloride prescription medications?

Notes:

37. Who is eligible to receive Chlorpromazine Hydrochloride prescription drug help?

Notes:

38. How do Chlorpromazine Hydrochloride prescription drugs work?

Notes:

39. Will my gender or ethnic group be denied Chlorpromazine Hydrochloride medications that work better for other groups but not for my ethnic or gender group?

Notes:

40. Who is at risk for Chlorpromazine Hydrochloride prescription drug addiction?

Notes:

41. When in care who is responsible for the MAR (Medication Administration Records), who can put information on to it and make changes?

Notes:

42. Who is validating my Chlorpromazine Hydrochloride prescription drugs to make sure I am taking the correct pills?

Notes:

43. What herbs, supplements, foods, drinks or activities should I avoid while taking Chlorpromazine Hydrochloride medication?

Notes:

44. Will Chlorpromazine Hydrochloride prescription medications cause gum problems?

Notes:

45. Who typically uses Chlorpromazine Hydrochloride prescription drugs, and where do they get them?

Notes:

46. Is there a Chlorpromazine Hydrochloride prescription drug guide on the internet?

Notes:

47. Am I up to date on my routine health maintenance?

Notes:

48. Who gets to see the Chlorpromazine Hydrochloride prescription drug information submitted in my patient medical questionnaire?

Notes:

49. Are Chlorpromazine Hydrochloride medications effective?

Notes:

50. Who makes this Chlorpromazine Hydrochloride medication?

Notes:

51. Is Chlorpromazine Hydrochloride a slow releasing medication?

Notes:

52. Who can get Medicare Chlorpromazine Hydrochloride prescription drug coverage?

Notes:

53. May my employer ask me which Chlorpromazine Hydrochloride prescription medications I am taking?

Notes:

54. How long am I expected to take this Chlorpromazine Hydrochloride medication?

Notes:

55. Is there anything I should do to help prevent my health issue?

Notes:

56. I take daily prescription medications, may I take my pills before I have my blood drawn?

Notes:

57. If I am unable to comply with the treatment regimen, who else can administer Chlorpromazine Hydrochloride medication?

Notes:

58. Can you slow down and keep it simple?

Notes:

CHAPTER #2: WHAT:

INTENT: What do I need to know about Chlorpromazine Hydrochloride (What will it do for me and what can I expect.)

1. What is the test for?

Notes:

2. What is the easiest way to obtain the latest information about Chlorpromazine Hydrochloride prescription drugs?

Notes:

3. What's the probability that my Chlorpromazine Hydrochloride medication is causing my symptoms?

Notes:

4. Can you help me understand how much of my Chlorpromazine Hydrochloride prescription drugs, equipment and services will be covered by my insurance and what I will have to pay?

Notes:

5. What types of vitamins and supplements should I be taking?

Notes:

6. What can I do to help win the war on prescription drug abuse?

Notes:

7. What happens if I stop using Chlorpromazine Hydrochloride cold-turkey?

Notes:

8. What types of Chlorpromazine Hydrochloride medications are available?

Notes:

9. What happens if I have to cut my Chlorpromazine Hydrochloride pills in half to make them last longer or skip a day of medication because I can't afford to buy it as often as it's prescribed?

Notes:

10. What would you do if you were me?

Notes:

11. What would happen if I don't take the Chlorpromazine Hydrochloride, would my health get worse?

Notes:

12. What is the safest way to dispose of unused prescription Chlorpromazine Hydrochloride medication?

Notes:

13. What are my options if I have difficulty paying for Chlorpromazine Hydrochloride prescription drugs?

Notes:

14. What should I do if I have other prescription drug coverage and want to join Medicare First?

Notes:

15. How will I benefit from working out in relation to my use of Chlorpromazine Hydrochloride prescription medication, and what type of exercise would you recommend?

Notes:

16. Is treatment required, if so - what is it?

Notes:

17. What about side effects of Chlorpromazine Hydrochloride?

Notes:

18. What are my Chlorpromazine Hydrochloride medication options?

Notes:

19. What kind of medication will I have to take, Chlorpromazine Hydrochloride or anything else?

Notes:

20. What if I am unhappy with the results of Chlorpromazine Hydrochloride medication?

Notes:

21. What about my regular medications, any interference with Chlorpromazine Hydrochloride?

Notes:

22. What are the causes of Chlorpromazine Hydrochloride prescription drug abuse?

Notes:

23. What medications are available to treat my condition?

Notes:

24. What does a Chlorpromazine Hydrochloride medication error involve?

Notes:

25. What is the evidence for this treatment?

Notes:

26. What Chlorpromazine Hydrochloride medications are used?

Notes:

27. What sources can I trust?

Notes:

28. How will you know what medications I am on?

Notes:

29. I want to read more about my condition. What online sources should I trust?

Notes:

30. What are the important warnings for males taking Chlorpromazine Hydrochloride?

Notes:

31. What really works as well as these Chlorpromazine Hydrochloride medications, are there alternatives?

Notes:

32. What kind of experience with these issues do you have?

Notes:

33. What is are food or drinks you recommend not to be taken with Chlorpromazine Hydrochloride prescription medications?

Notes:

34. What is the way to get my life back on track, without the unwanted side effects of Chlorpromazine Hydrochloride prescription drugs?

Notes:

35. What Chlorpromazine Hydrochloride medication should I take?

Notes:

36. What does my Chlorpromazine Hydrochloride medication look like?

Notes:

37. What other drugs could interact with Chlorpromazine Hydrochloride medication?

Notes:

38. What should I expect after a procedure in terms of soreness, what to watch for, Chlorpromazine Hydrochloride medication, bathing, and level of activity?

Notes:

39. What are your thoughts on hypnotherapy and Chlorpromazine Hydrochloride?

Notes:

40. What will a positive result mean?

Notes:

41. What's your go-to question for your own doctor?

Notes:

42. What is the prescription drug of choice for breakthrough pain meds?

Notes:

43. What else can I do to treat my condition?

Notes:

44. What is the proper course of treatment for me?

Notes:

45. What's the best mix for me of home remedies, over the counter (OTC) drugs and ointments and Chlorpromazine Hydrochloride prescription drugs?

Notes:

46. What happens if I don't do anything?

Notes:

47. What outcome should I expect?

Notes:

48. What are the important warnings for females taking Chlorpromazine Hydrochloride?

Notes:

49. What about taking a new Chlorpromazine Hydrochloride medication?

Notes:

50. What side effects can Chlorpromazine Hydrochloride medication cause?

Notes:

51. What is the name of my condition, are there any other names it's known by?

Notes:

52. What prescription medications or off the shelf medicinal products would cause ringing in the ears?

Notes:

53. What can I do to remember to take my Chlorpromazine Hydrochloride medication?

Notes:

54. What are the adverse health effects from Chlorpromazine Hydrochloride prescription drugs?

Notes:

55. What should I do if I experience side effects from the Chlorpromazine Hydrochloride?

Notes:

56. What are the Chlorpromazine Hydrochloride medication side-effects?

Notes:

57. What prescription drugs are you yourself taking?

Notes:

58. What medications can Chlorpromazine Hydrochloride interact with?

Notes:

59. In what way can mindfulness or meditation be useful?

Notes:

60. What to eat, or what to use as a medication together with Chlorpromazine Hydrochloride?

Notes:

61. What do I need to know about making the most of this Chlorpromazine Hydrochloride prescription?

Notes:

62. What exactly leads one to get dependent on Chlorpromazine Hydrochloride prescription drugs?

Notes:

63. What if I have been taking Chlorpromazine Hydrochloride medication with little to no relief?

Notes:

64. What causes my condition?

Notes:

65. What are the benefits of having the test?

Notes:

66. What is Chlorpromazine Hydrochloride prescription drug detox?

Notes:

67. What are my risks of accidentally taking an overdose of Chlorpromazine Hydrochloride prescription drugs?

Notes:

68. What if Chlorpromazine Hydrochloride medication has changed since the application form was sent in?

Notes:

69. What are the dosages of the Chlorpromazine Hydrochloride medication?

Notes:

70. What is the branded prescription drug fee?

Notes:

71. What are my options in relation to Chlorpromazine Hydrochloride medication, surgical procedures or remedy?

Notes:

72. What kind of expectations should I have?

Notes:

73. What will be the net effect of Chlorpromazine Hydrochloride medications for me?

Notes:

74. What Chlorpromazine Hydrochloride-like medications are safe to take during pregnancy?

Notes:

75. What kind of Chlorpromazine Hydrochloride medications do the varying plans offer and how much can I save?

Notes:

76. What if I have tried various home remedies, over-the-counter medications or even Chlorpromazine Hydrochloride prescription medications with no help?

Notes:

77. What is a 25/50 percent Chlorpromazine Hydrochloride prescription drug plan?

Notes:

78. What lifestyle changes can change my condition?

Notes:

79. What will happen if I don't have the treatment?

Notes:

80. What should I do if I miss my regular dose of Chlorpromazine Hydrochloride?

Notes:

81. What if I am currently taking some other prescription medications?

Notes:

82. What will happen to me without Chlorpromazine Hydrochloride prescription drugs, diet, exercise, or nutritional supplements?

Notes:

83. What could be a natural alternative to more over-the-counter and Chlorpromazine Hydrochloride prescription drugs?

Notes:

84. Is Chlorpromazine Hydrochloride safe when breastfeeding, what are the effects on nursing?

Notes:

85. What is my outcome?

Notes:

86. What is the effect of Chlorpromazine Hydrochloride on infertility?

Notes:

87. What are the signs and symptoms related to Chlorpromazine Hydrochloride addiction?

Notes:

88. What other Chlorpromazine Hydrochloride-like medications are in this class?

Notes:

89. What non-Chlorpromazine Hydrochloride medications or vitamins should I take to speed up my healing?

Notes:

90. What can I do to prevent my condition from recurring or worsening?

Notes:

91. What sort of Chlorpromazine Hydrochloride prescription drug benefit is included?

Notes:

92. What are the side effects of the Chlorpromazine Hydrochloride medication?

Notes:

93. What medications have you yourself used in the past to make yourself better?

Notes:

94. What is my Chlorpromazine Hydrochloride prescription drug benefit?

Notes:

95. What can parents and other adults do to help prevent prescription drug abuse among youth?

Notes:

96. Will I need medication and what will it be, Chlorpromazine Hydrochloride and/or anything else?

Notes:

97. Besides Chlorpromazine Hydrochloride medication, what else to do?

Notes:

98. What is the brand name for the drug Chlorpromazine Hydrochloride?

Notes:

99. What if I'm already on medication and have side-effects from the Chlorpromazine Hydrochloride?

Notes:

100. What is a generic Chlorpromazine Hydrochloride medication or drug, what does that term mean and what can it do for me?

Notes:

101. What's the difference between all of the Chlorpromazine Hydrochloride's class medications?

Notes:

102. What are other treatment options?

Notes:

103. What does this sign on my Chlorpromazine Hydrochloride prescription drug imply?

Notes:

104. What about Chlorpromazine Hydrochloride's interactions with my medications?

Notes:

105. What do you recommend to do with Chlorpromazine Hydrochloride medication adherence being difficult for me since my busy life pulls me in multiple directions - can you help me understand the ramifications of non-adherence?

Notes:

106. How do I book in to have the test and what is the usual waiting period?

Notes:

107. Apart from Chlorpromazine Hydrochloride medication, what are other components of your management plan?

Notes:

108. What will this test tell us?

Notes:

109. What is the nature of the Chlorpromazine Hydrochloride medications prescribed?

Notes:

110. What about alcohol and its effect on Chlorpromazine Hydrochloride prescription drugs?

Notes:

111. What if the Chlorpromazine Hydrochloride medications produce unwelcome or harmful effects?

Notes:

112. What if I'm taking other medication?

Notes:

113. What about Chlorpromazine Hydrochloride prescription drug coverage?

Notes:

114. What kind of resources do I have available to me?

Notes:

115. What about my current medications or allergies and the effect on it of Chlorpromazine Hydrochloride?

Notes:

116. At what point would you recommend Chlorpromazine Hydrochloride prescription drugs, alternative therapies, or surgery?

Notes:

117. What medications should I ask for?

Notes:

118. What's next?

Notes:

119. What is the name of my Chlorpromazine Hydrochloride medication?

Notes:

120. What sexual response side effects can I expect from these Chlorpromazine Hydrochloride medications?

Notes:

121. What Chlorpromazine Hydrochloride's class medication can I take best?

Notes:

122. What is the effect of Chlorpromazine Hydrochloride on drowsiness?

Notes:

123. Do I need to change what I eat or stop any Chlorpromazine Hydrochloride medications before doing a test?

Notes:

124. Is it possible that my employer may look at what Chlorpromazine Hydrochloride prescription medications I'm taking?

Notes:

125. For what reasons would I have to be off Chlorpromazine Hydrochloride medication and for how long?

Notes:

126. What Chlorpromazine Hydrochloride prescription drugs have serious side effects?

Notes:

127. What else could I be doing to stay healthy and prevent disease?

Notes:

128. What is the best approach if I forget to take this Chlorpromazine Hydrochloride medication?

Notes:

129. What are the side effects?

Notes:

130. What is the safest way to dispose of unwanted medications?

Notes:

131. What if my prescription Chlorpromazine Hydrochloride medication is lost or stolen?

Notes:

132. What if Chlorpromazine Hydrochloride medication makes me gain weight?

Notes:

133. What are some of the best non prescription medications I can give a try?

Notes:

134. What is Chlorpromazine Hydrochloride medication for?

Notes:

135. What can I expect from Chlorpromazine Hydrochloride medication?

Notes:

136. What should you, as my doctor, know before

prescribing Chlorpromazine Hydrochloride
medication?

Notes:

137. What if I take Chlorpromazine Hydrochloride
prescription drugs and get little or no relief?

Notes:

138. What will my Chlorpromazine Hydrochloride
medication do for me?

Notes:

139. What's to lose by trying another Chlorpromazine
Hydrochloride class medication?

Notes:

140. What happens with my prescriptions for
Chlorpromazine Hydrochloride medications while I
am travelling overseas, how to get and fulfil those?

Notes:

141. What are the different treatment options?

Notes:

142. What is a prescription drug error and how often and why do these errors occur??

Notes:

143. How do scientists determine whether the chemical compounds in Chlorpromazine Hydrochloride prescription medications do what they're claimed to do?

Notes:

144. What are your experiences with Chlorpromazine Hydrochloride prescription drugs?

Notes:

145. What is a generic Chlorpromazine Hydrochloride medication?

Notes:

146. What are good reasons to not take my Chlorpromazine Hydrochloride prescription medication?

Notes:

147. What replacement medications can you suggest for Chlorpromazine Hydrochloride?

Notes:

148. What medications on the market, OTC or Chlorpromazine Hydrochloride prescription, can become harmful over time and would be dangerous if used well past the expiration date?

Notes:

149. What other prescription drugs should I avoid while taking my Chlorpromazine Hydrochloride medicines?

Notes:

150. In what situation would I need to go for counseling if I'm receiving medication treatment?

Notes:

151. What are the Chlorpromazine Hydrochloride medications I can take?

Notes:

152. What if I have an allergic reaction to Chlorpromazine Hydrochloride?

Notes:

153. What other sources are available, who can I talk to about this?

Notes:

154. What should I know about Chlorpromazine Hydrochloride medication?

Notes:

155. What questions haven't I asked that I should have?

Notes:

156. What will a negative result mean?

Notes:

157. What if I am taking vitamins or over-the-counter drugs that could affect my Chlorpromazine Hydrochloride prescription drugs?

Notes:

CHAPTER #3: WHERE:

INTENT: Where to next (Where can I find more information. Do i need a second opionion. What happens with tests.)

1. Should I take medication to lower my blood pressure?

Notes:

2. If remedies help, what is the nature of Chlorpromazine Hydrochloride medications and where could one go to explore them?

Notes:

3. Should I stop my Chlorpromazine Hydrochloride medications before any procedure?

Notes:

4. Did you wash your hands?

Notes:

5. Where can I buy Chlorpromazine Hydrochloride prescription drugs cheaper?

Notes:

6. Is there an alternative medication?

Notes:

7. Can using too much or too little Chlorpromazine Hydrochloride prescription drugs harm my health?

Notes:

8. Will you try and keep my Chlorpromazine Hydrochloride medications at a level where I can function?

Notes:

9. If there is an all new Chlorpromazine Hydrochloride medication that comes up how can it have been adequately tested in terms of it's long term negative effects?

Notes:

10. Can anyone get these Chlorpromazine Hydrochloride prescription drugs?

Notes:

11. Do I really need this test?

Notes:

12. Which Chlorpromazine Hydrochloride-like medication gives the most rapid relief?

Notes:

13. Where are others buying their Chlorpromazine Hydrochloride prescription medications?

Notes:

14. Do I need any Chlorpromazine Hydrochloride medications?

Notes:

15. Would increasing the dose of Chlorpromazine Hydrochloride have a positive effect or would I be better off asking you to try some new medications?

Notes:

16. How to take Chlorpromazine Hydrochloride medication?

Notes:

17. Are there other remedies, is there any relief other than Chlorpromazine Hydrochloride Medication?

Notes:

18. Does Chlorpromazine Hydrochloride medication work?

Notes:

19. Are generics available for all Chlorpromazine Hydrochloride prescription drugs?

Notes:

20. Is it true that an online pharmacy can save me money on Chlorpromazine Hydrochloride prescription drugs?

Notes:

21. Is it normal to feel this way?

Notes:

22. Can I ever be free of having to use prescription drugs?

Notes:

23. Can natural be just as potent, if not more potent than over-the-counter drugs, creams and ointments?

Notes:

24. Will taking Chlorpromazine Hydrochloride medication effect my mission call?

Notes:

25. Has anyone ever used this Chlorpromazine Hydrochloride medication?

Notes:

26. Is it okay to take my Chlorpromazine Hydrochloride prescription drugs and multivitamin during a fast?

Notes:

27. Where can US citizens buy their prescription drugs online from legally, in confidence, and under which conditions?

Notes:

28. What f I have any allergies to food, medications or things in the environment?

Notes:

29. Where can I get my Chlorpromazine Hydrochloride prescription medications filled?

Notes:

30. Do you offer treatment programs for those suffering from Chlorpromazine Hydrochloride prescription drug addiction?

Notes:

31. Is the Chlorpromazine Hydrochloride medication safe?

Notes:

32. If I have been taking the same prescription drugs for a long time, when is it time to evaluate?

Notes:

33. Are my Chlorpromazine Hydrochloride medications safe to use while breastfeeding?

Notes:

34. How do I avoid getting in a place where I need so many prescription drugs to function?

Notes:

35. Will my body get to depend upon a certain amount of my Chlorpromazine Hydrochloride prescription drug, an amount that grows higher the longer I am on the drug?

Notes:

36. Should I take Chlorpromazine Hydrochloride with food or drink?

Notes:

37. How do I use my insurance to get discounts on my Chlorpromazine Hydrochloride prescription medication?

Notes:

38. Where would you send your partner or children?

Notes:

39. Can the nurse see me?

Notes:

40. Where would I store my Chlorpromazine Hydrochloride medications?

Notes:

41. Do you earn bonuses based on performance?

Notes:

42. Is it likely to get worse, or is it likely to get better?

Notes:

43. Are there simpler - safer options?

Notes:

44. Can I share Chlorpromazine Hydrochloride prescription drugs?

Notes:

45. Can my child have his or her Chlorpromazine Hydrochloride medication administered during the school day?

Notes:

46. Are there less intrusive, harmless and effective solutions instead of Chlorpromazine Hydrochloride prescription drugs?

Notes:

47. I Googled my symptoms and read this. Is it accurate?

Notes:

48. Are Chlorpromazine Hydrochloride prescription medications included in my monthly insurance fee?

Notes:

49. Where should I get my Chlorpromazine Hydrochloride prescription drugs?

Notes:

50. What is the safest prescription drug disposal method?

Notes:

51. Can Chlorpromazine Hydrochloride medications or my health problems keep me awake?

Notes:

52. Can you inform me about nutrition, exercise, Chlorpromazine Hydrochloride medications and complications?

Notes:

53. What are the best ways that do not require prescription medications to fall asleep faster?

Notes:

54. Where can I get more info about that?

Notes:

55. How will the treatment effect the medications that I currently take for _____?

Notes:

56. Where can I find info about taking more than one prescription medications together with Chlorpromazine Hydrochloride?

Notes:

57. Where do I go if I've run out of money and desperately need Chlorpromazine Hydrochloride medication or a medical procedure?

Notes:

58. Are medication reminders only for prescription medications?

Notes:

CHAPTER #4: WHEN:

INTENT: When should I take or stop taking Chlorpromazine Hydrochloride and how (When should I take it, stop taking it and how.)

1. Is there an effective herbal alternative or supplement to Chlorpromazine Hydrochloride medication?

Notes:

2. What are generic alternatives for my Chlorpromazine Hydrochloride prescription drugs?

Notes:

3. When and how will I get the results?

Notes:

4. Do you have research you can share on Chlorpromazine Hydrochloride prescription drug prices?

Notes:

5. Do you know of any natural medication to help?

Notes:

6. When should I be on Chlorpromazine Hydrochloride medication?

Notes:

7. Are my prescription drugs also available in a generic version?

Notes:

8. When will I know that I am taking excessive pain medication?

Notes:

9. What medications do I need to stop and when?

Notes:

10. Will I require any Chlorpromazine Hydrochloride prescription drugs?

Notes:

11. Do vitamins interact with Chlorpromazine Hydrochloride medications?

Notes:

12. Can and should I continue my Chlorpromazine Hydrochloride medication while on a weight loss diet?

Notes:

13. Are Chlorpromazine Hydrochloride prescription drugs covered?

Notes:

14. When should I stop taking Chlorpromazine Hydrochloride medication?

Notes:

15. Can Reiki be used when taking Chlorpromazine Hydrochloride medications?

Notes:

16. When should I stop using Chlorpromazine Hydrochloride medication because of....?

Notes:

17. Chlorpromazine Hydrochloride is most definitely a prescription drug?

Notes:

18. Will my Chlorpromazine Hydrochloride prescription drug have a drivers warning on it?

Notes:

19. What is the effect of my Chlorpromazine Hydrochloride use if I smoke?

Notes:

20. What does one do when the only real help, the only Chlorpromazine Hydrochloride medication available, no longer works?

Notes:

21. How do prescription medications compare to herbal forms of treatment for my condition?

Notes:

22. What is this Chlorpromazine Hydrochloride medication for, why am I taking it?

Notes:

23. Are herbal supplements safe when I am taking other Chlorpromazine Hydrochloride prescription medications?

Notes:

24. When does this Chlorpromazine Hydrochloride medication expire?

Notes:

25. Will grapefruit affect my Chlorpromazine Hydrochloride medications?

Notes:

26. Is Chlorpromazine Hydrochloride a medicine with real evidence?

Notes:

27. Can people be guilty of DUI if they are driving under the influence of Chlorpromazine Hydrochloride prescription medications?

Notes:

28. Is there anything I can do to improve it myself?

Notes:

29. If you have a Chlorpromazine Hydrochloride prescription drug in your pocket, outside of the container when arrested is that considered DUI?

Notes:

30. When is it appropriate and safe to prescribe Chlorpromazine Hydrochloride medication for my condition?

Notes:

31. Can enzymes be taken with other Chlorpromazine Hydrochloride prescription medications?

Notes:

32. When should I take this Chlorpromazine Hydrochloride medicine?

Notes:

33. When could Chlorpromazine Hydrochloride medication not be working anymore?

Notes:

34. Is this normal or should I see a shrink for Chlorpromazine Hydrochloride medication?

Notes:

35. Are any medications I am taking dangerous for my stage of this disease?

Notes:

36. When did you graduate from medical school?

Notes:

37. When does Chlorpromazine Hydrochloride medication begin working?

Notes:

38. What treatments, therapies and medications are recommended or available for my condition?

Notes:

39. Is it all right for me to take allergy medication?

Notes:

40. Can my condition come back?

Notes:

41. When might herbal and nutritional therapies be a good alternative to over-the-counter and Chlorpromazine Hydrochloride prescription medications for people with my condition?

Notes:

42. Which of my medications cause the most weight gain?

Notes:

43. Will I get possible side neuritis of Chlorpromazine Hydrochloride medications?

Notes:

44. Can I travel to _____ with prescription drugs used as medication for my condition?

Notes:

45. Is it either / or when it comes to natural medicines and Chlorpromazine Hydrochloride prescription drugs?

Notes:

46. When I have been on the same amount of Chlorpromazine Hydrochloride medication for years – when should that be re-evaluated?

Notes:

47. How and when should I take my Chlorpromazine Hydrochloride medication?

Notes:

48. What are some great ways to help remind me when to take Chlorpromazine Hydrochloride medications?

Notes:

49. How do I deal with any Chlorpromazine Hydrochloride prescription medication when a side effect may be stated as 'may cause nausea or vomiting'?

Notes:

50. When you prescribe Chlorpromazine Hydrochloride prescription medication for my condition, how do you weigh the side effects?

Notes:

51. Are there any known Chlorpromazine Hydrochloride prescription medication and chia seeds side effects when they are combined?

Notes:

52. I am paid to _____ for a living, will my performance improve or decrease while using Chlorpromazine Hydrochloride prescription drugs?

Notes:

53. Can a Chlorpromazine Hydrochloride prescription drug card preserve me cash?

Notes:

54. Where can one undertake Chlorpromazine Hydrochloride prescription drug addiction treatment?

Notes:

55. When can seniors join a Chlorpromazine Hydrochloride prescription drug plan?

Notes:

56. Do I need to see any other health professionals - such as specialists - physiotherapists - dieticians or dentists?

Notes:

57. How/when do I get test results?

Notes:

58. Does it matter at what time I use my Chlorpromazine Hydrochloride medication?

Notes:

CHAPTER #5: WHY:

INTENT: Why do I need Chlorpromazine Hydrochloride (Are there Alternatives. Why do I need it. Which symptoms does it medicate.)

1. Are there any co-pays for medical treatments, hospitalization or Chlorpromazine Hydrochloride prescription drugs?

Notes:

2. Will I have to take my medications forever?

Notes:

3. Can I take Chlorpromazine Hydrochloride with prescription medication or with an underlying medical condition?

Notes:

4. Why would I, while regularly taking prescription medications, have to approach grapefruit consumption with caution?

Notes:

5. Why is this Chlorpromazine Hydrochloride medication prescribed?

Notes:

6. Is _____ a side effect of Chlorpromazine Hydrochloride medication and is it permanent?

Notes:

7. What if my religion condones the use of Chlorpromazine Hydrochloride medications?

Notes:

8. Why are you doing this test?

Notes:

9. What does using a prescription drug Off-label mean?

Notes:

10. What do you turn to for adjunctive medications, usually?

Notes:

11. Are you aware of my personal medical history including current medications, allergies, and other considerations or limitations?

Notes:

12. Who monitors the safety and effectiveness of Chlorpromazine Hydrochloride prescription drugs?

Notes:

13. Will Chlorpromazine Hydrochloride have an effect on nausea?

Notes:

14. Have you heard any stories about buying Chlorpromazine Hydrochloride prescription drugs over the internet?

Notes:

15. Why and when use acupuncture for treating pain instead of, or combined with, taking pain medication?

Notes:

16. Will any of the supplements that have been prescribed for me interfere with any Chlorpromazine Hydrochloride prescription medications I may already be on?

Notes:

17. Why is it important to take my Chlorpromazine Hydrochloride prescription medication exactly as prescribed?

Notes:

18. What would happen if I were suddenly unable to get access to my Chlorpromazine Hydrochloride prescription drugs?

Notes:

19. Why does a prescription drug require authorization by a qualified professional and others do not?

Notes:

20. Is the answer in natural supplements, in Chlorpromazine Hydrochloride prescription medications or some combination of both?

Notes:

21. When is it time to think about why I'm on these Chlorpromazine Hydrochloride drugs?

Notes:

22. How long will I need to take this Chlorpromazine Hydrochloride medication?

Notes:

23. Are there generic equivalents available for my Chlorpromazine Hydrochloride prescription drugs?

Notes:

24. If I take a Chlorpromazine Hydrochloride medication, will it require more medication to counter the side effects?

Notes:

25. Why do I need to manage Chlorpromazine Hydrochloride medications?

Notes:

26. Why do I need Chlorpromazine Hydrochloride medicine?

Notes:

27. Can we really know what is in Chlorpromazine Hydrochloride prescription drugs?

Notes:

28. Will you try and reach the primary reason for my problem before prescribing Chlorpromazine Hydrochloride medications to solve my particular signs and symptoms?

Notes:

29. Why are Chlorpromazine Hydrochloride medications so popular?

Notes:

30. Why would I need Chlorpromazine Hydrochloride prescription medication reminders?

Notes:

31. Is sharing Chlorpromazine Hydrochloride prescription drugs illegal?

Notes:

32. Does my health insurance plan provide prescription drug benefits?

Notes:

33. Can I take Chlorpromazine Hydrochloride medication?

Notes:

34. Why does my family's medical history matter, and what should I do about it?

Notes:

35. What do each of these Chlorpromazine Hydrochloride prescription medications have in common?

Notes:

36. Why have my bowel habits/appetite/mood/sex drive/etc changed?

Notes:

37. Why are you giving me a blood test - and what will the results tell us?

Notes:

38. What are the differences between generic and brand medications?

Notes:

39. Are any nutrients depleted by this Chlorpromazine Hydrochloride medication?

Notes:

40. What exactly is this Chlorpromazine Hydrochloride medication for in my case and how do you think it is working so well?

Notes:

41. Why is buying Chlorpromazine Hydrochloride prescription drugs without a prescription dangerous?

Notes:

42. Why is Chlorpromazine Hydrochloride a prescription drug?

Notes:

43. Why is Chlorpromazine Hydrochloride medication prescribed?

Notes:

44. What if I refuse the prescribed Chlorpromazine Hydrochloride medication?

Notes:

45. Why can't I buy some prescription drugs online?

Notes:

46. Why are we doing these tests?

Notes:

47. Will I be able to do _____ after treatment?

Notes:

48. What does 50 deductible for brand name prescription drugs mean?

Notes:

49. Should I lock up my Chlorpromazine Hydrochloride prescription drugs?

Notes:

50. Why go the Chlorpromazine Hydrochloride medication route?

Notes:

51. Is Chlorpromazine Hydrochloride addictive?

Notes:

52. Can I schedule my surgery for the morning?

Notes:

53. Can all doctors prescribe Chlorpromazine Hydrochloride Prescription Medication?

Notes:

54. Are there any other precautions or warnings for this Chlorpromazine Hydrochloride medication?

Notes:

55. Which Chlorpromazine Hydrochloride prescription drugs can be addictive?

Notes:

56. Is Chlorpromazine Hydrochloride safe if taking medications for high blood pressure?

Notes:

57. Could I have afforded it without Chlorpromazine Hydrochloride prescription drug insurance?

Notes:

58. Can Chlorpromazine Hydrochloride prescription drugs cause problems during pregnancy?

Notes:

CHAPTER #6: HOW:

INTENT: How will Chlorpromazine Hydrochloride affect me (How will it affect me negatively. How do I know if its a problem for me.)

1. How can my mental state successfully improve using medication or therapy?

Notes:

2. Are there drugs to lift my mood, and how can this be achieved without prescription medications?

Notes:

3. How long does a Chlorpromazine Hydrochloride medication remain active in your body?

Notes:

4. How should I take this Chlorpromazine Hydrochloride medication?

Notes:

5. So how do I save money on my Chlorpromazine Hydrochloride prescription drugs?

Notes:

6. How can I reduce or stop some of my medications?

Notes:

7. How often is the Chlorpromazine Hydrochloride medication taken?

Notes:

8. So how do you know if you, or someone you love is having problems with Chlorpromazine Hydrochloride prescription drug abuse?

Notes:

9. How long do I need to take the Chlorpromazine Hydrochloride medicine for?

Notes:

10. How's my weight?

Notes:

11. How soon do I need to have the test?

Notes:

12. How are Chlorpromazine Hydrochloride prescription drugs abused?

Notes:

13. How accurate are the results of the test?

Notes:

14. How serious is this condition?

Notes:

15. How do I know if I have permanent hair loss due to medication?

Notes:

16. How does a person with dementia, living alone, manage her Chlorpromazine Hydrochloride medication?

Notes:

17. How do different Chlorpromazine Hydrochloride-class prescription medications work differently?

Notes:

18. How will I hear about my test results?

Notes:

19. How wide-ranging is the Chlorpromazine Hydrochloride prescription drug coverage?

Notes:

20. How long will it take to get the results?

Notes:

21. How will I know if my current Chlorpromazine Hydrochloride Prescription Drug coverage is as good as the new Medicare Chlorpromazine Hydrochloride Prescription Drug coverage?

Notes:

22. How about a new Chlorpromazine Hydrochloride-like prescription drug?

Notes:

23. How do I read the label on my Chlorpromazine Hydrochloride prescription drug package?

Notes:

24. How can I make sure I am sufficiently stocked with the Chlorpromazine Hydrochloride prescription

medications I need?

Notes:

25. How do generic medications compare in quality to brand name drugs?

Notes:

26. How do I take this Chlorpromazine Hydrochloride medication?

Notes:

27. How is the test done?

Notes:

28. How effective is this treatment?

Notes:

29. How can I find a few methods that can help my condition without the use of Chlorpromazine Hydrochloride prescription medication?

Notes:

30. How should this Chlorpromazine Hydrochloride medication be taken?

Notes:

31. So I got a condition and a Chlorpromazine Hydrochloride medication – how am I, as a patient, supposed to manage treatment?

Notes:

32. State prescription drug price web sites, how useful are they to me as a Chlorpromazine Hydrochloride consumer?

Notes:

33. How should I use this Chlorpromazine Hydrochloride medication?

Notes:

34. How to go about it if I want to use a lower dosage of Chlorpromazine Hydrochloride?

Notes:

35. How do I manage multiple prescription medications together with Chlorpromazine Hydrochloride?

Notes:

36. How can I support my bone health naturally with and without medication?

Notes:

37. How is the Chlorpromazine Hydrochloride medication delivered?

Notes:

38. How can I reduce my Chlorpromazine Hydrochloride prescription drug costs?

Notes:

39. How can Chlorpromazine Hydrochloride prescription drug abuse be recognized and stopped?

Notes:

40. How often do I need to have the test done?

Notes:

41. How often will I take the Chlorpromazine Hydrochloride medication?

Notes:

42. How should this Chlorpromazine Hydrochloride medication be stored?

Notes:

43. How long will I need the treatment for?

Notes:

44. Is it probable to find out how to deal with my condition without taking Chlorpromazine Hydrochloride prescription drugs?

Notes:

45. How quickly do I have to start the treatment?

Notes:

46. How long does the Chlorpromazine Hydrochloride medication last?

Notes:

47. How do you handle children on Chlorpromazine Hydrochloride medication?

Notes:

48. Do you know how long it will take me to get my Chlorpromazine Hydrochloride medication?

Notes:

49. How many patients with my condition have you treated?

Notes:

50. How does Chlorpromazine Hydrochloride prescription drug abuse start?

Notes:

51. How can Chlorpromazine Hydrochloride medication be detected?

Notes:

52. How do I get better without Chlorpromazine Hydrochloride medication?

Notes:

53. How long do I have to take Chlorpromazine Hydrochloride medication?

Notes:

54. How do I dispose of Chlorpromazine Hydrochloride prescription medications?

Notes:

55. Are there support groups for people with this problem and how would I contact them?

Notes:

56. How should I dispose of Chlorpromazine Hydrochloride prescription drugs?

Notes:

57. How will Chlorpromazine Hydrochloride affect the other medications that I'm taking?

Notes:

58. My Chlorpromazine Hydrochloride medications, just how safe are they?

Notes:

59. How soon should I come back?

Notes:

60. How will I know if the Chlorpromazine Hydrochloride prescription and over-the-counter

medications I take are interacting properly?

Notes:

61. How is Chlorpromazine Hydrochloride medication supposed to help me?

Notes:

62. How long should I take Chlorpromazine Hydrochloride medication?

Notes:

63. How can I opt for the generic alternative Chlorpromazine Hydrochloride medication that gives me the exact same results?

Notes:

64. How do I manage my Chlorpromazine Hydrochloride medications?

Notes:

65. How can I dispose of my Chlorpromazine

Hydrochloride prescription drugs safely?

Notes:

66. How does Chlorpromazine Hydrochloride interact with other medications?

Notes:

67. How to store Chlorpromazine Hydrochloride medication?

Notes:

68. How do we order or pick up Chlorpromazine Hydrochloride medications?

Notes:

69. How many surgeries do you perform each year?

Notes:

70. How can I learn more about my symptoms or condition?

Notes:

71. How will I get the test results?

Notes:

72. How will Chlorpromazine Hydrochloride affect my sleeping pattern?

Notes:

73. How should I take my Chlorpromazine Hydrochloride medication?

Notes:

74. In case I need pain relief, how can I get access to medical cannabis?

Notes:

75. How long is it likely to last?

Notes:

76. How long does the prescription drug Chlorpromazine Hydrochloride stay in your system?

Notes:

77. How do the police suspect impairment by Chlorpromazine Hydrochloride prescription medication?

Notes:

78. How will I feel when I'm on Chlorpromazine Hydrochloride medications?

Notes:

79. How common is Chlorpromazine Hydrochloride prescription drug abuse?

Notes:

80. How long will the effect of Chlorpromazine Hydrochloride medication last?

Notes:

CHAPTER #7: HOW MUCH:

INTENT: How much will taking Chlorpromazine Hydrochloride cost me (In money and Chlorpromazine Hydrochloride's effect on quality of life.)

1. Do I need this particular Chlorpromazine Hydrochloride medication?

Notes:

2. Are there any side effects from taking nutritional supplements and Chlorpromazine Hydrochloride prescription medications at the same time?

Notes:

3. How much experience with this test or procedure do you have?

Notes:

4. Will kinesiology interfere with Chlorpromazine Hydrochloride medication?

Notes:

5. Will Medicare be enough to cover the cost of my medical care, especially Chlorpromazine Hydrochloride prescription drugs?

Notes:

6. Am I am worrying too much?

Notes:

7. Should I have a current emergency contact form and a list of health conditions and medications readily available?

Notes:

8. Is this necessary now?

Notes:

9. How much can I use this Chlorpromazine Hydrochloride prescription drug plan?

Notes:

10. Is this something I should worry about or is it just a side effect of Chlorpromazine Hydrochloride?

Notes:

11. Is switching from one biologic medication to another effective?

Notes:

12. How much should I be charged for my Chlorpromazine Hydrochloride prescription medications?

Notes:

13. Is Chlorpromazine Hydrochloride a medication?

Notes:

14. How much does Chlorpromazine Hydrochloride cost?

Notes:

15. Are there any side effects associated with this Chlorpromazine Hydrochloride medication that I should know about?

Notes:

16. Where does my Chlorpromazine Hydrochloride prescription medication come from?

Notes:

17. Will the cost be covered by Medicare - my concession or Veterans Affairs card or by private health insurance?

Notes:

18. Will Chlorpromazine Hydrochloride interfere with other prescription medications?

Notes:

19. What if my current Chlorpromazine Hydrochloride prescription drugs are not on the formulary or are limited on the formulary?

Notes:

20. Regarding dosage, exactly how much of Chlorpromazine Hydrochloride can I take?

Notes:

21. How much will this cost me?

Notes:

22. What are the Chlorpromazine Hydrochloride prescription drug prices?

Notes:

23. How do I know how much my Chlorpromazine Hydrochloride prescription medication will be?

Notes:

24. Common side effects of Chlorpromazine Hydrochloride include?

Notes:

25. Is there a better way to easily adhere to Chlorpromazine Hydrochloride prescription medication regimens?

Notes:

26. How do I get the Medicare Chlorpromazine Hydrochloride prescription drug benefit?

Notes:

27. How much will the test cost?

Notes:

28. If I need a surgery and I did go ahead with the surgery, how might that affect the Chlorpromazine Hydrochloride medications I take?

Notes:

29. How much will it cost, will the cost be covered by the PBS - my concession or Veterans Affairs card or by private health insurance?

Notes:

30. Which part of Medicare will cover my Chlorpromazine Hydrochloride prescription drugs?

Notes:

31. How much Chlorpromazine Hydrochloride medication can be brought through customs in case I travel?

Notes:

32. Are these Chlorpromazine Hydrochloride medications really helping?

Notes:

33. How much Chlorpromazine Hydrochloride prescription medication can I order from my pharmacy at one time?

Notes:

34. Please explain, what are the differences between generic and brand Chlorpromazine Hydrochloride medications?

Notes:

35. Can you suggest alternatives to Chlorpromazine Hydrochloride prescription medication?

Notes:

36. Is it covered by Medicare - my concession or Veterans Affairs card or my private health insurance?

Notes:

37. How much do I need to really understand about the interactions of my Chlorpromazine Hydrochloride prescription drugs?

Notes:

38. I feel like I need more medication, will you as my doctor be able to support me with my requests?

Notes:

39. Is there a Medicare Advantage plan provider who will cover my Chlorpromazine Hydrochloride prescription drug costs during the donut hole?

Notes:

40. Do pill boxes help prevent Chlorpromazine Hydrochloride medication errors?

Notes:

41. What prescription drugs do I need covered?

Notes:

42. How much is Medicare Chlorpromazine Hydrochloride prescription drug coverage worth?

Notes:

43. Just how much do you know about the numerous types of Chlorpromazine Hydrochloride medications for the different types of my condition?

Notes:

44. Can nutritional yeasts, especially brewers yeast, interact with Chlorpromazine Hydrochloride medications?

Notes:

45. Should I join a Medicare Prescription Drug Plan even if I don't take many prescription drugs?

Notes:

46. Should I rely on Chlorpromazine Hydrochloride, natural cures or over the counter medication?

Notes:

47. How much am I likely to spend on Chlorpromazine Hydrochloride prescription drugs?

Notes:

48. How much does it normally cost to get the surgery done, including all Chlorpromazine Hydrochloride medications and tests (ultrasounds,x-rays,medicines, hospital stay)?

Notes:

49. How much will my Chlorpromazine Hydrochloride prescription drugs cost me?

Notes:

50. How much will the treatment cost?

Notes:

51. How much will the plan cover for Chlorpromazine Hydrochloride prescription drugs?

Notes:

52. Are there medications available that really fix the underlying cause of my condition?

Notes:

53. Do we have to do this test now?

Notes:

54. Are there any other medicines that can help me but without any side effects?

Notes:

55. Are there health insurers who reimburse for Chlorpromazine Hydrochloride prescription drugs based on how well they work?

Notes:

56. If I am taking Chlorpromazine Hydrochloride prescription medications can I take natural remedies?

Notes:

57. How much do the Chlorpromazine Hydrochloride prescription drugs cost in this plan as compared to other plans?

Notes:

58. Can you explain my options for Medicare, Medicare/Medicaid, Disability, Supplemental Insurance, Part D Prescription Drug Plans, or Medicare Billings?

Notes:

Index

possible   44, 73
potent 56
precaution   1
precise 1
pregnancy   34, 89
prepare   4
prepared   5
prescribe   1, 71, 75, 88
prescribed   22, 41, 79, 81, 87
prescribes   3
preserve   75
pressing   4
pressure   52, 89
prevent   9, 18, 37-38, 45, 116
prices 66, 112
primary   84
private 111, 114-115
proactive   3
probable   99
problem   5, 84, 91, 102
problems   9, 16, 62, 89, 92
procedure   27, 52, 63, 108
procedures   3, 34
process   3
produce   42
product   1, 3
products   1, 11, 30
programs   58
proper 28
properly   103
provide   84
provider   116
providers   3, 5
provides   5
providing   3
publisher   1
purchase   3
purchased   3
qualified   12, 82
quality 3, 96, 108
question   2-3, 6, 28
questions   3-5, 50
quickly 100